HOW TO LOSE BELLY FAT FAST

For Men and Women

EMMA GREEN

Book
3

CONTENTS

Foreword	v
Introduction	ix
1. U.S. Obesity Statistics	1
2. The Real Science of Belly Fat	6
3. Exercise, Weight Loss, and Why You Struggle	11
4. The 6 Cup A Day Rule	18
5. Foods and Drinks to Avoid	24
6. The PH Balance of Food Is Paramount	31
7. Chrysanthemum Flowers Are Truly Amazing	34
8. The Miracle of the Ancient Practice of Stomach Rubbing	40
9. Boost the Loss with Bike Riding	44
10. Eight Great Green Smoothie Recipes for You to Enjoy!	47
In Conclusion	53

FOREWORD

"I love everything about Emma's connection to weight loss and health."

Hi, my name is Nat Lee, and I've spent most of my life looking pretty good and feeling great. That was up until I started eating on the run and allowing my busy life as a mom to take hold of me. While working too.

In truth, I knew I should eat great food, but time constraints and "motherly craziness" got the better of me. I made sure my son ate well. But I didn't, which was silly, really. Parenting is one of those things that just takes over your life, I suppose. So, anyway, I kinda ate loads of stuff I shouldn't, and drank sodas and milkshakes an awful lot. Chocolate and takeout became my best friend, and I became overweight, by anyone's standards. No one really told me I looked bad, I mean, most people aren't that obvious. But when I was diagnosed with a severe illness and bedridden for four years, it became time to do something to help my recovery. I made the change as soon as I could.

Since reading Emma's books, I've lost 18.5 kg (which is 40 amazing pounds). And I've managed to keep it off by following her wonderful advice, and by using her awesome, easy-to-do recipes. I live relatively simply, but her guide to nutrition and her tips and tricks have helped me a bucket load. Thank you Emma, you've literally changed my life!

© Copyright 2017 - All rights reserved.

In no way is it legal to reproduce, duplicate, or transmit any part of this document in either electronic means or in printed format. Recording of this publication is strictly prohibited and any storage of this document is not allowed unless with written permission from the publisher. All rights reserved.

The information provided herein is stated to be truthful and consistent, in that any liability, in terms of inattention or otherwise, by any usage or abuse of any policies, processes, or directions contained within is the solitary and utter responsibility of the recipient reader. Under no circumstances will any legal responsibility or blame be held against the publisher for any reparation, damages, or monetary loss due to the information herein, either directly or indirectly.

Respective authors own all copyrights not held by the publisher.

Legal Notice:

This book is copyright protected. This is only for personal use. You cannot amend, distribute, sell, use, quote or paraphrase any part or the content within this book without the consent of the author or copyright owner. Legal action will be pursued if this is breached.

Disclaimer Notice:

Please note the information contained within this document is for educational and entertainment purposes only. Every attempt has been made to provide accurate, up to date and reliable complete information. No warranties of any kind are expressed or implied. Readers acknowledge that the author is not engaging in the rendering of legal, financial, medical or professional advice.

INTRODUCTION

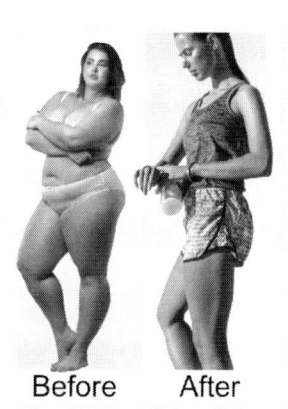

Before   After

Hi! Thanks so much for meeting me here in this title. I can't wait to share all my knowledge with you, so you too; can get the body you want. And, just so you know, I always promote doing this in safety, and with great health as the most important aspect. Because YOU are really important!

My name is Emma Green, and I lost over 100 pounds in 22 months! As it turned out, I had been doing everything back-to-front and upside down. I had been exercising without paying attention to my diet or any nutritional needs at all. I'd tried multiple brands of "skinny" pills, and I had been riding a stationary bike for hours on end (with marginal results). I tried everything... Yep! I even starved myself with diets that gave temporary results. The stress of doing all of it with little to no results made me feel absolutely hopeless, worthless, and more than overly annoyed! Many times, I felt like completely giving up. I was lost and felt like I couldn't find my way out of it. I nearly gave up! Semi-depressed was my state of mind. It felt like everything sucked. I was very sad, mad, and exhausted. And then my aunt had a stroke, and (god-willing) she survived. But, from that point on, and after suffering severe arthritis, I made an effort to change.

Oh, let me remind you, if you haven't already read my mega title, "How I Lost 100 Pounds! My Personal Weight Loss Strategies for Optimum Happiness," make sure you get your FREE copy today. Inside you'll learn exactly how I lost my weight, and the benefits of knowing the must-do nutrition, and other amazing secrets including myths, water weight, the only exercise you really need, the ancient and easy technique to help slim you quickly, how to balance meals, and much, much more! I hope you love it. It's my very special gift to you!

There are a vast number of people who lead healthy lives, but they are still faced with a continual problem area of their body. This is not to say they are overweight, but sometimes they just can't remove those few extra pounds that sit around their middle - no matter how hard they try.

There are reasons this happens, and how to tackle the problem can be seen through the following chapters, and also via the issue of dietary confusion and a lack of knowledge on how to do it. I didn't really know where to turn when I made the choice to lose weight. This is why I'm writing this title.

I want to take the time to congratulate you on your efforts to change yourself, because, in reality, just taking the time to do that takes strength and loads of foresight, so I am here cheering you on. I absolutely feel that I can help you on your journey, because, I myself, did this too.

In truth, I know that there are loads of books sharing tips and tricks to do this... but I know this works, because I absolutely know what it takes to get there, and I have lost over 100 pounds. I also know how tough losing weight can be if you never get shown how to do it. So, let's get started together. Remember, I am here the whole way through, with you. And yes, I'm definitely supporting you right throughout your entire journey. Please know how much I want this for you!

So, let's get started, and see what we can do. Chapter 1 will start with the sad statistics that are overshadowing America, presently. Globally, they are catching up, too. I think these points are necessary, to be both a backbone for motivation and to widen our knowledge basis as a whole. Let's go!

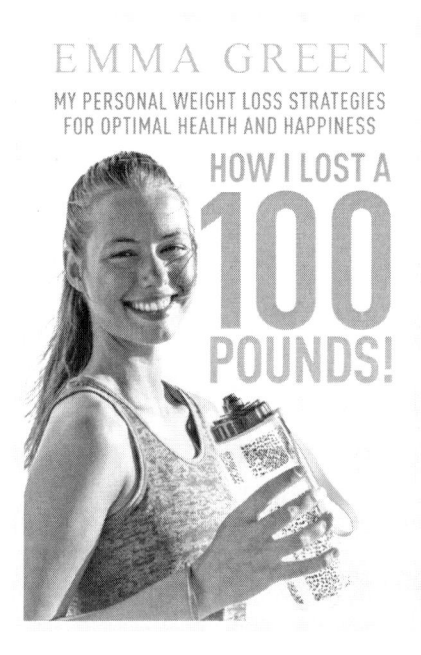

Btw check out "How i lost a 100 pounds" if you haven't already, its got loads of value and its completely FREE :)

FREE GIFTS!

Here are 3 bonus books I want to gift you for coming and reading this title! Sign up to my newsletter and you will receive:

Weight Loss Myths - 9 myths that you are mostly likely doing right now that are totally pointless and are a waste of time toward your weight loss goals.

How to Lose Weight Fast – A 10 day plan I personally put together to make that weight literally melt before your eyes (it worked for me!)

And... Weight Loss Secrets - Secrets the main stream media and health industry never talk about because (let's be honest) things that work don't make them money!

Click here to sign up! or for paperback versions grab it through the ebook completely FREE!

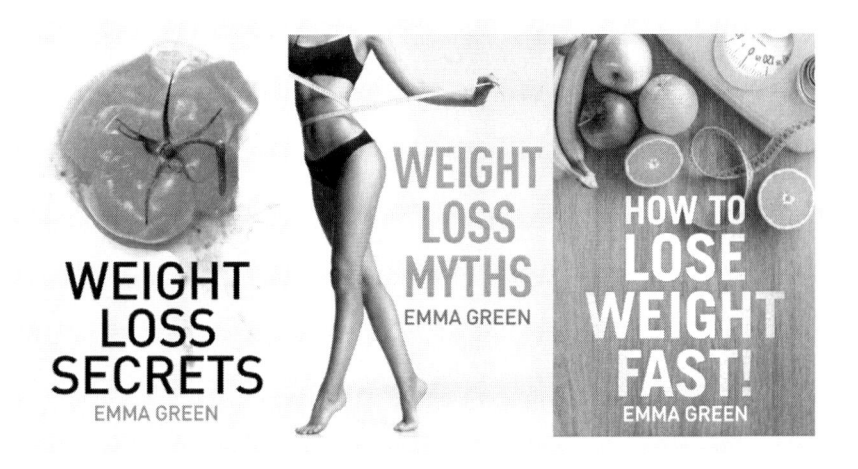

Chapter One
U.S. OBESITY STATISTICS

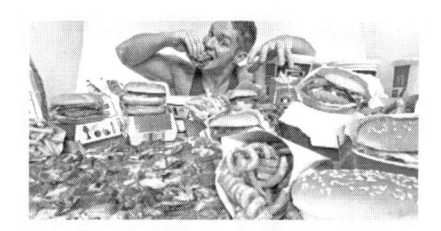

Many of the country's officials have a significant concern about the epidemic that is sweeping the country of America. It is so much of a problem that around 70% of the county officials who were asked, have, in fact, ranked it as one of the leading issues in the area that they reside in.

This epidemic is obesity, and it is not only hitting adults, but there are also a vast number of children of varying ages who are also being tremendously affected. The concern among officials is that if this trend continues, the youth of today might just be the first generation that starts to live shorter lives and be (overall) less-healthy than their parents.

Studies show the problem with obesity varies throughout the states, yet it is consistently high, and now it is showing us that: **one in three adults, and one in six children between the ages of 2 and 19 years of age, are obese.**

The range for adults is from the lowest state (which has a little over 22% obesity) to the highest state (that has just over 37% of an obesity problem). **It should be noted that in over 20 states, unfortunately, these obesity rates show up at a rate of over 40% in some counties.**

When these individuals are exposed to these sorts of weight problems, they become exposed to a significant risk in: type 2 diabetes, dementia, some forms of cancer, and heart disease, to name a few. In the cases of obesity in children, it is more likely that they will carry this condition over into their adult lives, so these illnesses are more likely to hit them as they get older, too.

What is more alarming than these figures, is the numbers that are rising of individuals with extreme obesity, and this figure is higher in women than it is in men. Currently, the percentage of women who are extremely obese is around 10% while men are a little over 5%, so it is almost double. When the figure for extreme obesity is taken as an average for the country, it is just under 8% of the current statistics that have been published in recent times.

Obesity Trends

Since 1980, the statistics for children in the age group for 12 to

19 years has quadrupled from 5% in 1980, to 20.5% in more recent years.

For children that are younger (and in the age group of 2 to 5 years old), almost 10% are classed as obese with 2% being extremely obese.

When the figures for adults are analyzed, they show that in 1985 not one state had a rate of obesity over 15%. In 1991, the next round of numbers showed no state had an obesity problem of over 20%. Later, in 2000, no states reported a value of 25%. It was only six years later the first state reported numbers of over 30% obesity in adults. And it has been climbing ever since.

When age groups in adult figures were recently studied, **it showed that 40-59-year-old adults have a 41% obesity problem when compared to the 20-39-year-olds who have a 34% obesity problem. For adults of 60 and over, the percentage was 38%.**

While these studies were conducted, it was shown that between the years 2008-2010, that almost 33% of adults who never graduated from high school had an obesity problem. This was compared to a figure of 21.5% of individuals who graduated from a technical college or a college. This bears some relation to the figures which showed at the same time: 33% of adults who earned less than $15,000 per year found they suffered from obesity, whereas the number for individuals who earned above $50,000 per year was 24.6%. I, personally, believe the link to be a lack of knowledge. And it is the most unfortunate thing to see. Because, in truth, if the knowledge is shared widely, then we could educate everyone. This, regardless of any social, political, economic, educational, racial, gender, (or any other) standing in society.

Financial Costs of Obesity

As a nation, **more than $150 billion is spent on healthcare each year.** For obesity, the figures run into billions - and an estimated value of **$6 billion per year is lost due to indirect absenteeism at work or children in schools from the problem.**

It has also been shown, that the number of individuals who are able to serve as first responders, including police officers and firefighters (or even military personnel) has diminished due to this problem. These are not the only costs or losses that are attributed to the obesity epidemic. These figures do not include the many hundreds of millions of dollars that are used to fund science into obesity and a way that the U.S. can tackle the problem.

This epidemic has spanned for over three decades, and all the industries, foundations, and government agencies who have contributed these funds into the fight against obesity have spent skyrocketing amounts. They have funded and conducted clinical trials, major studies, and the development of drugs that are all geared toward quashing the rise of obesity. But drugs to fix a problem that can be prevented is a whole other title. We won't go there, today.

Even after all this time, and after all the resources that have gone into these studies, the rise of obesity shows no sign of diminishing anytime soon. Some of the onus might be pushed onto the establishments who provide the means of putting food onto the Americans' table to help with this fight. But, until then, the figures look even worse for the future. The Center for Disease Control and Prevention predict that: in another ten years the number of individuals who suffer from obesity will be around 42%, while The Trust for America's Health gives figures of approximately 44%. Wow, that's astonishing, and something needs to change.

Individuals can help, and that is what this book hopes to address. A lot of the problem comes from easily accessible processed foods. For years, people have battled with being overweight, and **over $20 billion is spent in America on slimming products alone.** Many of these are done by "get rich quick" companies who are taking advantage and, in reality, do nothing to contribute to the problem, even though they promise a... "New, healthier you."

Taking the matter into your own hands can make all the difference. And, after all, who wants to be just another statistic? Let's go! We've totally got this!

Chapter Two

THE REAL SCIENCE OF BELLY FAT

After seeing the statistics from Chapter 1, hopefully you are more determined to try and lose those few extra pounds from around your waist, and it's definitely worth mentioning why they are there in the first place. This is especially true if the remainder of your body is generally in good shape.

Quite a few people fall foul to this around holiday periods, especially toward the later parts of the year. First up is Thanksgiving, with only a few weeks before Christmas and New Year's. This is the time that a lot of Americans pile on those pounds that they are then unable to shift easily.

With lots of larger meals, including holiday parties with drinks and the extra snacks that are consumed, an average American can easily gain an extra two pounds in weight. With this, it is unfortunate that most of it ends up around the abdomen area.

If this problem is not tackled as soon as the holidays are over, this weight can become a permanent fixture, and you are probably already aware, it is the hardest part of your body to get back into shape.

The Science Behind Those Extra Pounds

It's important to understand how your body reacts to this influx of festive foods and the complex science that comes behind any weight loss. Here, you will see how the body stores these stubborn fat deposits, and what it is using that fat for.

Storing fat in the body is a factor that ensures survival. It has been this way all throughout the many centuries of evolution. It started from the very first days and was nature's way of protecting the body during food shortages. Although we have evolved by countless thousands of years, and it is rare to go for extended periods without food and becoming hungry, **the human body still has this defense mechanism.** And so, it processes food in much the same way as it has always done. It likes to make us survive.

In modern day society, it is a general way of life to eat more and to exercise less than our ancestors did all those years ago. Quite a bit of this can be substantiated by the statistics we saw earlier, and that show the increase in obesity since the 1980s. To amplify the problem today, it is not only how much we eat, it is the types of foods we eat that make things definitively worse.

The body now has to cope with many more types of foods and drinks than were available to our ancestors, and now we can take a look at how and where the body stores this fat - and how it processes it.

Fat and Energy

It is a real shame that things have gone the way they have, because, in truth, **fat is a fantastic source of energy when burned as fuel for the body**. If you take a look at junk foods, these are very high in fat and they leave you unsatisfied and hungry once the initial burst of gratification has been felt. This leads to the problem of overeating, and in many cases, this would be more junk food. This cycle can continue with an ever-increasing intake of fat with little to no chance of it being burned as energy.

Fats are also known by the name "triglycerides," and when these are consumed they are broken down by the body and passed around the bloodstream. It is at this stage they are burned as energy (or stored as fat reserves) for future use.

When this fat is ingested, it actually becomes stored into fat cells by the name of adipocytes, and these cells are located all around the body under the layer of skin with a high number of them deposited in the abdominal region of the body - unfortunately.

So, when this fat is not burned for energy, it is stored continually until the time when the body needs energy reserves. If a current state of overeating and lack of exercise ensues, then this leads to an inactive lifestyle which then leads to the body's metabolism becoming slower. And so, there is less requirement for it to burn these fat deposits.

Two Types of Belly Fat?

There are, in fact, two types of fat around the midsection. The first is **visceral** which surrounds our internal organs and the second is **subcutaneous** which is that podge that we love to grab and squeeze! Well, that we "used to" love to grab and squeeze.

Now, with these two fats, the one that surrounds the organs is visceral, and it's actually the one that is easier to deal with. This can be rectified by a healthier diet and taking up exercise. Subcutaneous fat is the type that causes the most problems and is the one that is most difficult to lose. It is this one that leaves us with the unflattering "love handles" and "beer bellies" that so many adults are blessed with.

A Vicious Circle

If it was just these that caused problems, it might be easier to cope with and reduce those extra pounds around the belly. But... nature has one more surprise up its sleeve for all the dieters out there.

When the body is stressed, hormones are released from the adrenal glands. These being cortisol, norepinephrine, and epinephrine. When you first become stressed, that's when it's time for these hormones to come into play.

Norepinephrine passes signals to the body to halt the production of insulin, and so you can have a larger supply of fast-acting blood glucose for when it is needed. Next, epinephrine relaxes the muscles in the abdominal region muscles and intestines while (at the same time) reducing the blood flow to these. Once the stressor has passed, it is the job of cortisol to tell the body to stop these other two hormones being produced, and return to its normal functioning and digest again, normally.

In a regular day, your cortisol levels will vary and can rise and fall. If you become continually stressed your cortisol levels can rise and remain at this level. If you are stressed and cortisol remains at this higher level, then the body can actually resist any attempts at weight loss. It is this in-built trigger that relates stress to the past state of survival as a necessity, where times were harder, and food was in short supply. And so, the body hoards what it can to preserve its energy reserves.

The body (when in this state) can do one of two things, it takes the fat you consume, or it can take fat from other healthy parts of the body and move it toward your abdominal area which contains more of these cortisol receptors.

This is what makes it harder to lose these pounds, because the more stressed you get about it, the more the body tries to put fat around your waist. If that wasn't enough, these peripheral fat deposits that were somewhat healthy are converted into visceral fat that surrounds the organs, **it is this chronic buildup that leads to illness and inflammation, along with insulin resistance in the body.**

Now a vicious circle can start, because this belly fat leads to an increase of cortisol due to a higher concentration of the enzyme which will convert inactive cortisone into active cortisol. Now, the cycle continues, and more enzymes equals more fat, which again, equals more enzymes, and yes, you have guessed it... more fat.

Although there is actually quite a lot of science behind it, you can see why the stomach gains fat first, and loses it last. This knowledge is great to know, because if we understand this, we can do something about it! And that's why we're here.

Chapter Three

EXERCISE, WEIGHT LOSS, AND WHY YOU STRUGGLE

When trying to lose weight, everyone has always been taught to do plenty of exercise, and if you have a few extra stubborn pounds around your waistline, you might have been tempted to put even more effort in to try and shift them.

Now, in hindsight, it has come to light that this approach might be all wrong and that it could actually be hurting weight loss, for several reasons. This basically means there is a correct way to go about losing weight and that, without knowing this, it might make weight loss more difficult.

Here are a few reasons why you might not be losing weight as you expected (no matter what you do), exercise wise:

The Wrong Foods

I did this lots. Fried chicken, sugary biscuits, and cakes were my loves. We all know eating junk foods is not healthy, and there are many foods that we consider good. And they are, in fact, making weight loss around the belly that bit more difficult. **A healthy diet makes up 80% of the weight loss battle rather than more exercise.** Wow, huh?

Any foods that are starchy should be reduced, and the amounts of protein in your meals should be increased (more on this in the next chapter).

You Are Probably Eating Too Much

I did this too. Actually, eating the "wrong" foods will make you overeat because they are mostly high GI. Giving you a blast of energy and then making you crave more of the same. If you are struggling to lose belly fat and you have reduced your intake, it might be the case that you are still overeating without realising. You might have already cut lots out, but everyone's bodies and lifestyles are different, and so, you might need to reduce more calories to help shift those last few pounds. It should be noted that this does not mean you have to starve when you choose the "right" healthy foods, and you will feel fuller for longer, so you will have less temptation to snack between meals.

If you feel you are deprived when it comes to food, then that's one of the reasons people slip and binge which negates all the hard work they have already done.

Too Much Cardio

Exercise makes up 20% of the weight loss program, and it does keep you healthy and fend off disease and illness. And here, your metabolism increases, and it helps you to break out into a good sweat. You should break out into a good sweat daily, because this helps with water retention (explained later).

Cardio has been seen as the best way to fight the flab, yet too much can aid the problem. If you eat healthily and are doing lots of cardio-type exercises, your body can be eating away at lean muscle mass rather than the fat deposits around your waste. This muscle mass is vital because it is this that burns calories when your metabolism increases.

Secondly, all this **cardio will increase appetite** and will leave you more tempted to snack or overeat. We don't want that. The other thing to stress, is that your heart can be placed under too much pressure with too much exercise. We want to help health, not negate it. Some might argue differently, but many studies show that too much is not good. We need balance, always.

Lifting Weights

To make sure your body does not slip into this endurance-focused mode and tries to preserve itself some energy, you should ditch some of the cardio and lift a few weights. This has a couple of advantages. The first is, that it **helps to maintain or build up your lean muscle mass** that is all-important for burning calories. The more muscle tone you have around the body, the more fat you can burn. **It's a symbiotic relationship.**

Not Working the Right Way

As each and everyone's body is different, there is no set rule of how much exercise you should be doing in relation to what you are eating. This could take some experimentation to find a balance that is good and perfect for you.

As mentioned above, more work in the gym is not necessarily the answer, so it is wiser to get your healthy eating in check before committing to hitting the gym for ridiculous workouts each and every week. You really don't need to. And there is one major exercise that's best for targeting the area of the belly. We will explain this later on!!

One pound of weight equates to 3500 calories which you need to burn. So, if you reduce calories by a set amount you will naturally lose weight, albeit slowly.

To get by, an average sized woman needs to consume 2000 calories per day, and an average working male needs 2500 calories per day. **If you reduce your intake to: a minimum of 1200 calories, per day (for women), and 1700 (for men), you can lose 5600 calories per week** - which would equate to 1 1/2 lbs. per week in natural weight loss. Wow!!

When it comes to your exercise, we know too much cardio can have an adverse effect. Workouts should be shorter rather than longer, yet the work you do should be more intense, and this gives the benefit of the **"afterburn"** effect which keeps your metabolism at a raised level for between 24-48 hours afterword, and without harming your lean muscle mass.

Recovery Time

Do light exercise that is enough to keep you burning calories. Even housework or mowing the lawn can help! And although the recommended exercise per day is 30 minutes to maintain fitness, no one should be working out for more than one hour per day. This is true, especially when they're trying to achieve weight loss.

Sleep and Weight Loss

When I was at my heaviest, I found myself tossing and turning most nights. I did all the right things, and even counted sheep, sometimes. I think the pain from my arthritis kept me up a little, but as I lost weight my sleep improved by volumes. It was like the best possible cure for insomnia, ever!

Even my boss at the time noticed that I looked "more alive" at work, as he stated. And he even told me he'd been beginning to worry about me. Thankfully, I managed to fix my problem, but there are loads of people who have this issue; it's really draining. Losing weight changed everything for me. Sleep patterns, energy levels, and my self-esteem.

The importance of enough sleep can also come into play with regard to increased cortisol levels. If you don't get enough sleep then these levels can rise, and they'll show up in the following evening from when the sleep deprivation occurred. In recent times, many **Americans are reporting less sleep on a regular basis,** and this gives even more insight into why weight problems are so widespread.

Lack of sleep can also have an effect on hunger levels which relates to two hormones called leptin and ghrelin. **Leptin tells the body when it is full, and it is the function of ghrelin to send out signals for hunger.** Even with just two nights where sleep has been reduced, there can be an increase in the amount of the hunger hormone (ghrelin) and a reduction in the amount of leptin (satiety) levels in the blood.

This leads to show us just how important sleep really is. So, make sure you are able to get sufficient sleep, otherwise your body will be receiving lots of mixed up signals. And we want balance in all ways. **Balance creates harmony and healing, which can help the body**

to achieve weight loss. Stress relief is also a major factor, and nutrition.

Increasing Carbohydrates

There is one other thing to consider when it comes to balancing your exercise with the foods you eat. Overall, a reduction in carbohydrates is one of the best types of foods to reduce when looking to lose weight. However, **for workout days it is better to increase carb intake because a lower carb intake has the effect of raising cortisol levels in the body.** White rice is my carbohydrate of choice. It aids the body in digestion too.

Exercise Stress

In the previous chapter, it was mentioned what role stress has on the body. It forces it into a self-preservation mode and pushes fat into the abdominal region. **Exercise is a stressor on the body, and unfortunately, the body is unable to tell the difference between stress from exercise and stress from work, as an example.** And, if it feels stress, the body then kicks into self-preservation mode and tries to push fat cells toward the stomach. Oh no! We don't want that, do we?

This was the cycle I was in, and for months on end! It drove me crazy until I learned I was overdoing it.

When you eat healthily and have a healthy balance of non-stressful exercises, your body will not try to produce these high amounts of cortisol for extended periods of time.

Now, we can see that excessive exercise on a daily basis can harm your efforts in reducing those pounds around the belly, and we now know why they are so stubborn to move. So, utilize less time exercising, with a more beneficial type of exercise (we'll cover this soon), and a healthier way of eating. This is all a major part of the secret to losing weight more naturally – especially belly fat.

Chapter Four

THE 6 CUP A DAY RULE

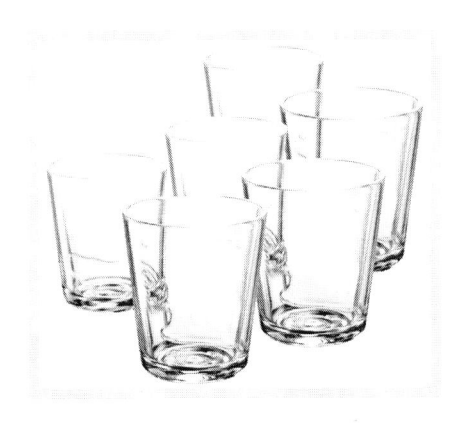

This was the real kicker for me. I would drink and drink until the cows came home... I love that expression. But seriously, I was keeping the weight on (water weight) because I'd learned to. "My mom would say, "Make sure you drink plenty of water." And that expression and mode of thinking gets handed down from generation to generation. It is totally wrong. Let's see why...

While you are aiming to lose belly fat quickly, you will come to find that a lot of weight in the body is from excess water. With extra exercise and a higher intake of fiber, it is crucial to remain hydrated, but... **too many fluids can have an adverse effect on the body.**

The following advice is taken from Taoist teachings which have been around for thousands of years and have proven effective in helping the body function at its most optimum level, especially regarding fluids in the body and how they affect specific elements.

It is the function of the kidneys to filter waste from the blood and during the period of a day they can only filter a set amount. If there is an increase over this they can become overworked, and if they are strained for extended periods of time, they WILL become weaker, and in a worst-case scenario, they can actually fail.

When kidneys are healthy and performing at their most optimal, they can filter 6 cups of fluids (water or other liquids) in a 24-hour period.

Maintaining Fluid Levels

If you drink the **6 cups of fluids per day**, your body will sustain itself on a balanced level. If you drink more than this, your kidneys are unable to filter this excess, and the fluid remains inside the body and continues to travel around the bloodstream. It will then need to be eliminated through perspiration when exercising, or in hot weather, as another example.

Unfortunately, if you drink more than six cups per day, these fluids can remain in the body and will become an unwanted part of your excess weight. Even if the weather is hot and you exercise a fair amount, your body will only perspire part of this excess water that you consume. This leads to another problem which can be slightly harder to rectify.

What Happens to Excess Fluids in the Body?

When there are still excess fluids in the body which are not lost through perspiration, they start to sit under the layers of skin as they wait to be expelled as perspiration. As new fluids are introduced, this backup of fluid under the skin will increase, and the **skin becomes bloated** because it is readying itself to expel fluids through the pores. Unfortunately, it discharges as much as it can and the remaining fluids that continually backup become stagnant, and contain in them, the **numerous toxins and waste products** that should have been eliminated.

This builds up over time is considered the same as urine, and if too many fluids are sitting under the skin, they have the potential to remain there for days, weeks, or even years without being discharged. This is not good for health.

Over prolonged periods, this buildup of stagnant water turns into a substance similar to thick mucus, yet, it is still water. There are many individuals who are none-the-wiser about the effect this excess water is having. Actually, they think they are carrying around extra fat, although there is a chance it is this mucus that is trapped between the muscles and tissues that they have a problem with.

From the stages of this mucus-like liquid, a further hardening occurs inside the body, and this transforms into what we know as **cellulite.** This can form on parts of the body where perspiration will be at its least.

What to Do with Cellulite?

Anyone who has tried to lose weight knows that cellulite is a problem to get rid of. Much of this problem comes from the fact that cellulite is not a fluid that can be expelled by conventional means, and it is not a body fat that can be removed by dieting and exercise, either.

There are ways you can tackle this cellulite problem. And, when coupled with **the keto/paleo diet styles** and a healthy exercise plan, it can help individuals to lose belly fat, fast. The part of being able to address this cellulite problem is to **limit your intake of fluids to 6 cups per day.** This ensures you will not have a buildup of fluids that will only aggravate the problem. This is, in fact, the essential part of the cellulite removal process, and without doing this, as hard as you try - you will not notice any major reduction.

The second part of the process is to break up these cellulite deposits, so that they can be eliminated by the body more easily. This can be done using **hot baths or saunas** and then you may break down the deposits using a **massage.**

In layman's terms, the more you work on these deposits, the more they can be broken down, and with the effects of a sauna or hot bath, the pores are opened wider and can allow for more perspiration.

What's in 6 Cups?

Because this problem is from fluids (and not one of overeating), many people follow a diet and have salads, soups, or even smoothies. And this is awesome. In one way they are doing the right thing, yet regarding cellulite, they are not considering the amount of water that is in their meal/drink. **This should be included in your maximum of six cups per day.**

Calculating these fluid levels in hard foods can be difficult, and this is one of the beauties of juicing or drinking nutritious smoothies. Here, the foods are broken down into a near-liquid form, so what is measured is classed as part of your fluid intake for the day. This makes it easier to control, and it also makes it easier to know what you have remaining to reach the 6-cup limit.

How to Tell if you Have Water Retention?

Even if you do not have a cellulite problem, you might be carrying around excess water that you can get rid of to help with your belly fat loss. **One of the simplest ways to do so is to push your finger hard against the skin of your arm or your leg.** Once you remove your finger, you will see a mark, or you will see nothing at all. If there is no white mark remaining, it means you do not have a water retention problem, but if there is a mark that stays there for a second or two, then this is an indication that you have a problem. **The longer the mark remains on your skin, the larger the water retention is within the body.**

One word of advice is not to use diuretic tablets that are often prescribed by physicians. In truth, this places you in a never-ending loop of water weight issues. You take a diuretic tablet to remove excess fluid, yet you drink more, as advised. All this does is replace what was expelled, so the fluid levels never actually decrease.

It is more natural and way healthier to limit your fluids to 6 cups per day and it will reduce the strain on your kidneys, too. Additionally, you will automatically see the change after a week of doing so, or maybe earlier, depending on your individual body and its functioning.

This point is pivotal in any weight loss regime. And forever-after too. Tell everyone about it, because it can mean the difference between health and becoming very unwell.

Chapter Five
FOODS AND DRINKS TO AVOID

When it comes to food and weight loss, there are certain things to avoid altogether, and food items you should eat in moderation.

Although you might already have reduced calories, you could still be consuming more than you think. A wiser approach can be to look at your everyday habits which can cause weight gain, or which are preventing you losing those few extra pounds around your stomach. One of the secrets is knowing that going on a diet creates an obsession with food, and this actually heightens cravings because you feel you are deprived.

This can be the main reason that people quit on a diet and say it does not work. When you are reducing your calorie intake, it is crucial that you know how a small, "extra thing" can make a massive difference to your daily intake. **Good examples are: a spoonful of salad dressing that can quickly add up to 100 calories to your meal, while a spoonful of butter adds almost the same. A small bag of** chips that accompanies your lunch adds nearly 200 calories, which is a fair chunk of your daily allocation.

Aside from this, there are the regular foods you eat, and how they mount up, yet they do not do much to help you feel satiated. It is easy to fall into bad habits. When this happens, it is another thing that makes those last few pounds extremely challenging to remove.

A high number of individuals fall into bad habits when trying to lose weight, here are some of the most common:

Hectic lifestyles do not leave us much time to **eat at a leisurely pace**, yet this has been shown to be more beneficial, because it is easier to savor the food in front of you, and you get a greater sense of being full than when eating on the go.

Skipping meals is one of the leading bad habits and does nothing to help. When trying to lose weight, you should make sure you eat three meals per day. It has been shown that you'll consume fewer calories than you would by skipping a meal and making up for it later. Each meal should contain a portion of carbs, proteins, and fat, so you get a full range of nutrients and vitamins. You also need to eat three times a day at regular intervals, so that your blood sugar levels stay well-balanced.

Calories in drinks are the one area many people underestimate the calories being consumed. A study showed that an average American adult received around 21% of their calories from various types of beverages.

Foods to Avoid and Why

One of the first things to avoid is sugary drinks, and this is not only in the case of sodas and energy drinks. There are a high number of fruit juices which aren't great for you and that contain a large amount of calories, too. There is also the misconception that drinking fruit juices rather than eating a meal is good for you. We want balance, not starvation. So, don't do that, please.

Actually, **many fruits contain high amounts of natural sugars**. Drinking anything will never be a substitute for food when feeling hungry, as drinks deal with thirst, and not hunger. If you are to consume juices, it should be fresh vegetable juices which are very high in vitamins and nutrients, while still being low in calories. I will share some great green smoothie recipes at the end of this title.

High sugary and salty snacks are the types of food you should entirely avoid. This can include potato chips, popcorn that has been artificially flavored, ice cream, cakes, cookies, and candies. Not only are these full of calories, but the ingredients they contain might make you feel like eating more. There are loads of additives and "processes" which are not natural in these foods. So, avoid "junk" food, altogether.

Sugar-free products are one of the tricky ones. They might be low in calories, yet they contain artificial sweeteners which make you feel hungry and give you more cravings. So, in truth, they backfire the cause entirely.

Multigrain products should be avoided because they are only labeled this way to trick you into thinking they are healthy. Multigrain is a fancy name for products that are full of processed carbs. Just choose "whole grain" products if you are ever unsure.

Following on from multigrain is **white bread**, and it contains high amounts of added sugar and will spike your blood sugar levels. It's loaded with calories, too. I used to love white bread, but now I don't miss it at all.

Candy bars are conveniently placed everywhere and should be avoided at all costs. Even though they might be small, they are packed full of calories, added sugars, oils, and refined flours. They have no place in health, at all.

Store bought fruit juices should be avoided. As mentioned earlier, they are highly processed and full of added sugars. Unfortunately, they bear no resemblance to the fruits they are portrayed to containing. With no fiber, they require no chewing and have no effect on you feeling full, like you would with a fresh orange, for example. Juicing with real fruit is so much more beneficial.

Cakes, cookies, and pastries are made from highly refined flours and contain vast amounts of sugars. Many are also made using trans-fats which are harmful, and they are not very satisfying, and hunger will quickly return once you have eaten them.

Most types of **alcohol** contain more calories than both protein and carbs. Beer is the worst alcohol to drink, yet a glass of red wine with a healthy Mediterranean-type meal can be beneficial.

The list goes on for any **processed foods**, or foods that contain ingredients that are hard to pronounce. Yet all is not rosy on the fruit and vegetable side as you would expect. There are some (that although healthy) aren't very helpful when it comes to shifting those few pounds around the belly area.

Tropical fruits taste delicious, yet mango and pineapples contain more sugar than other fruits, and as an aside, they contain more calories too.

Dried fruits have more calories in smaller quantities, the only difference being they have had their water removed. If you consume these as a snack, you seriously have to limit yourself because of the moreish taste.

Mashed potato might seem healthy for many reasons, but they come with a large amount of calories when compared to equal weights of other foods. They also have a high glycemic index which spikes blood sugar levels. I use sweet potato because it's low GI. It gives the body energy over time. Pumpkin can also become a substitute here.

Other foods that might appear to be healthy and are not as healthy or nutritious as they seem. These should be avoided or consumed rarely and in small portions. They are:

Flavored Yogurts – Contains high amounts of sugar.

Granola – Labeled as healthy, yet full of sugars and fats.

Bagels – These contain the same amount of carbs as in 6 slices of white bread.

Pasta – Here, most of the goodness has been stripped in processing.

Coleslaw – Although most of it is cabbage and vegetables, that mayo covering it is loaded with calories.

Dairy – Full of protein and calcium, yet one small bite-sized cube of cheese can contain 70 calories. It is also highly acidic.

Deli meats – Deli meats are mainly processed, one example being salami, which is high calories.

Bottled Waters

Many people choose to drink bottled water rather than rain or filtered water. Most bottled tap water has no major benefit and is just put into fancy bottles before shipping it to market.

To make sure you are drinking pure water, **it is better to drink distilled water as this contains no impurities compared to other types of bottled waters.** How do you really know a bottled water's source?

Distilled water is as pure as water can get. In addition to this, another real misconception is that most nutrients come from the foods we eat and not from the water we consume. **The daily allocation of water only contains 15% of the daily organic content the body needs on a regular basis.**

Distilled water brings with it the advantage of eliminating poisons from the body. This is due to distilled water being efficient in removing toxins. Never drink tap water, because it is loaded with nasty chemicals, **including fluoride** which is not conducive to long term health when ingested.

Allen E. Banik, M.D. Author, "The Choice is Clear" wrote:

"Distilled water is the greatest solvent on earth. (It is) the only water that can be taken into the body without damage to the tissues.

What we as scientists and the public have never realized is that minerals collected in the body from water are all inorganic minerals, which cannot be assimilated (digested) by the body. The only minerals that the body can utilize are the organic minerals (from fruits and vegetables). All other types of minerals are foreign substances to the body and must be disposed of or eliminated."

He went on to say, "Today, many progressive doctors prescribe distilled water to their patients. All kidney machines operate on distilled water."

Here is what Dr. Teofilio de la Torre says...

"Instead of drinking the hard water of springs or the chlorinated water of the cities, it will be to our advantage to drink distilled water . . . to prevent calcification of the body."

Other harmful additives in tap water include: chloride, lead, mercury, arsenic, perchlorate, dioxins, fluoride, polychlorinated biphenyls, DDT (insecticide), HCB (a pesticide), dacthal, and MtBE. Some are more prevalent in certain countries than in others. It's like a horror story, really.

Chapter Six
THE PH BALANCE OF FOOD IS PARAMOUNT

The term having a "balanced diet" is said quite a lot when people are looking at losing weight or maintaining their own health promotion. It is a broadly used term, yet many people do not fully understand the meaning behind it. Many people would interpret this as making sure that you consume foods which belong to the primary four food groups.

Much of this comes from western nutritionists, but what they say is not the whole of the picture when it comes to food and its PH. And, more definitively, how it affects the body and your diet on the whole.

Rather than informing individuals of foods to eat from the four food groups, it should be the acids and alkalinity levels that are contained in foods that are advised, and how this affects your overall wellbeing.

In the Stomach

When foods reach the stomach, they are broken down and assimilated by the body. However, if they are too alkaline or too acidic, they are not digested as well as they could be. It is the case that when foods have a reduced PH and their acid-alkaline is out of balance, then these foods are allowed to decompose inside the digestive tract. As with any food matter that is allowed to decay, it becomes the ideal breeding ground for germs, parasites, and bacteria. All which enter the body by way of foods.

A Healthy PH

When a stomach has a healthy PH level, this helps to keep these germs and parasites from breeding, and then the body is allowed to metabolize the food correctly. When this PH is out of balance or missing, it will enable the food to become corrupted by microorganisms which reside in foods and inside the body. When this happens, the body (instead of reaping the benefits of the nutrients of the food) absorbs the poisons that are created from the corrupted foods.

For an example of what happens, you can look at the rear of any restaurant and see all the scraps of food that are decomposing in trash cans. Only a few hours before, this same food was being served to customers. With just a few hours of time difference, you can see what happens to these foods, and it is, in essence, the same as what is happening inside the stomach.

No one would even consider eating food (garbage) that was exposed to this environment, yet when there is no consideration for the PH in the foods we consume, this is precisely what we are doing without realizing it. So, yes, PH on an internal level is paramount.

A Balanced PH

One sign of an unbalanced stomach PH is actually bad breath, and if we begin to consider a food's PH and how the stomach can be balanced, then it makes sense. In reality, it can be passed quickly and efficiently through the digestive tract with no fear of decomposition and/or a buildup of parasites.

A regular diet for Americans consists of too many foods which are considered acidic while consumption of alkaline foods is negligible, to say the least.

Balancing your PH levels so that your cells can maintain homeostasis (the perfect balance for functioning and healing processes) is easy. The best rule of thumb is to eat 80% alkaline foods, each day. High alkaline foods include: broccoli, kale, parsley, spinach, radish, wheatgrass, alkaline water, sea salt, mineral salts, Himalayan salt, barley grass, herbs, spices, flaxseed oil, avocados, cherries, hemp hearts, chia seeds, quinoa, herbal tea, raw tomatoes, lemons, and limes.

White Rice is Beneficial

It's important to note the benefit of white rice as a staple food. It has been milled to eliminate the shell that forms around the seed. Brown rice has not had this process done, and so is harder for the body to chew, digest, and cook with. Brown rice is a good source of nutrition, but white rice is easier on the body and its processes. In fact, all nutrients can be absorbed easily when white rice is used in meals. The other important factor is that it will balance out any dish; complementing, neutralizing, and balancing it, completely. In this way, ulcers, heartburn and stomach issues can be prevented, according to Taiost theories involving the Five Tastes and the Five Element Theory. So very advised to always have rice with meals when possible.

Chapter Seven
CHRYSANTHEMUM FLOWERS ARE TRULY AMAZING

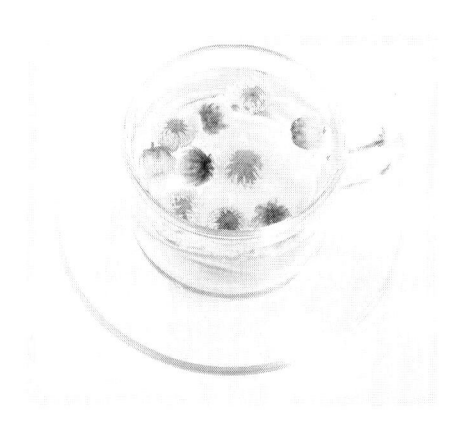

Chrysanthemums are common around the world and adorn many people's gardens. What has recently come to light is how beneficial they are to the human body. Such is their ability to give many health benefits; they have been used in Chinese medicine for thousands of years.

Scientific Studies

To test their properties, a test was conducted that used four groups of mice. The first group (A) was fed a high fat/cholesterol diet, and (B) was fed the same (yet with chrysanthemum flowers incorporated into their foods), as well. The third group (C) was fed a diet of low fat and cholesterol, while group (D) was fed the same, but with the chrysanthemum flowers added into the food.

When the results of the study became finalized, it showed that group (B) that was fed chrysanthemum flowers as part of their high fat and high cholesterol diet, showed reduced blood cholesterol levels. The numbers were so impressive that they almost matched group (D) that was fed a low-fat and low-cholesterol diet.

Chrysanthemum Tea

The easiest way to add chrysanthemum flowers to your diet is by way of drinking a tea made from them. Where this tea differs from others, is the fact that the full plant is used when brewing rather than only the flower of the plant.

When hot water is infused with the full plant, there are numerous antioxidants, nutrients, minerals, and vitamins that are released along with amino acids. The amino acids make it a highly nutritious and tasty tea that has an excellent soothing effect on the whole body.

Major Benefits of Chrysanthemum Flowers

Many benefits have been found when drinking this tea, and they can bring an overall sense of wellbeing, rather than only focusing on one type of ailment inside the body. When some of the benefits are grouped together, it is easy to see that they can help digestive problems and that they show an increase in assisting the body to regain healthier digestion, overall.

Chrysanthemum is full of flavonoids which have natural antioxidant properties which help prevent many health risks. They are shown to act as an anti-inflammatory which can reduce irritants throughout the body. This occurs along with having antibiotic effects that help to prevent the buildup of harmful bacteria in the body, as well as in the digestive tract.

Eye health can also be improved as this tea is packed full of Vitamin A and can help to reduce redness, dryness, and itchiness. As cholesterol levels are brought back into check, it goes a long way to promote heart health and lower blood pressure levels to help prevent further cardiovascular disease, as well. All of these benefits not only support health, but they aid in weight loss promotion too.

One of the primary uses that chrysanthemum tea has been used for over the years, has been as a natural treatment for the common cold and help to improve respiratory problems. This is achieved by strengthening the lungs and maintaining them in excellent, pristine condition.

Chrysanthemum tea (when consumed over extended periods) helps with blood flow and the effects of aging, and additionally, healthier skin is seen as an apparent result of this. Such was its relevance in Chinese medicine, and it was considered the favorite drink of a high number of Taoists.

Overall consumption of the tea helps to calm and soothe the body's nerves while aiding with the natural digestion functions of the body when taken as part of a healthy diet, and when taken with food. The foods it works so hard at neutralizing are greasy or deep-fried foods, which is why the scientific tests showed such good results for the mice who were fed a high-fat diet. The ones with chrysanthemum flowers included in their food.

Tea made from these flowers is also caffeine free, so it can be consumed throughout the day with no harmful effects, including the fear of palpitations, or being unable to sleep properly. If you utilize a keto-styled diet, the tea will most-definitely aid the body where weight loss is concerned. A natural helper, it seems. A great addition to your day.

Chapter 9: The Five Tastes and the Five Element Theory

What is not considered or advised upon in western medicine is the aspect of taste between foods. In Chinese medicine, it has been shown that taste plays a vital role in the foods we eat and therefore our body's processes, too. Fundamentally, the body is adversely affected by the theory pertaining to the groups and the percentages that are ingested by the individual.

What Are the Five Tastes?

The five tastes that we should eat as part of a healthy diet are known as: "**Sweet,**" twenty percent, "**Sour,**" twenty percent, "**Salty,**" twenty percent, "**Bitter,**" twenty percent, and "**Spicy,**" twenty percent.

Although all of these appear to be how foods will taste, and they also affect what they will do once they are inside the body. A prime example of this is the liver and gallbladder. When these detect a sour taste, they create bile, which helps your body to break down deep fried or greasy and oily foods. All of which are well known to hinder the function of the liver.

Five Tastes and Body Organs

In Chinese medicine, each of these five tastes is related to an area of internal organs.

Sweet is related to all the digestive organs which include the pancreas, spleen, and the stomach.

Salty is related to any water organs such as the bladder and the kidneys.

Sour as we have just seen, is related to the liver and gallbladder, while **Bitter** is related to the heart.

The **Spicy** taste is linked to the lungs and to the large intestine. These are the two major elimination organs that have the duty of ridding the body of waste, be it food, or air.

The pairings that come with organs and foods which are related to them are based on the reaction to taste and the way the organs function. And with this in mind, Chinese medicine aims to bring the body back into balance, and food is one of the most accessible ways to achieve and maintain this balance.

The Chinese have stated that when you are mindful and aware of these five flavors, you can go on to lead a long and healthy life. It is when we have too much of one taste and not enough of another, that this leads to disease or illness.

It is essential to eat the correct percentage of each taste throughout the day. There are many foods which consist of one flavor such as a banana, which is sweet. There are many foods which complicate things a little and have two tastes such as ginseng, which is both bitter and sweet. Another example is plums which can be both sweet and sour.

The five tastes are also linked to seasons of the year, so eating vegetables that are grown at that time can help to achieve the right balance, too.

Bitter is related to early midsummer, so vegetables like spinach, kale and bitter gourd (among others) are available at that time to help cleanse the body.

Salty relates to the winter season, so any foods help retain fluids when the season is dry. The salty taste is not meant to be from table salt which is full of chemicals, it is sea salt, sea vegetables, and natural soy sauce which helps to clear sinus passages, as an example.

Sweet relates to late summer. Their effect is aimed at relaxation and can include foods such as carrots, sweet potato, onions, corn, and cooked cabbage.

Sour is related to the spring where any sour tasting foods give a quick burst of energy. Citrus fruits such as berries, tomatoes, lime, lemon, and pickles can be used. Some enhance the appetite, while others make foods taste even more delicious.

Spicy (pungent) is related to autumn and can help the lungs and the intestines. However, too much of this can irritate the intestines. In most dishes, they are paired with foods high in fat because they help to break down plague accumulation in the body. Ginger, garlic, wasabi, and peppers help with the flushing out of toxins and wastes.

Chapter Eight
THE MIRACLE OF THE ANCIENT PRACTICE OF STOMACH RUBBING

This exercise is so simple to perform that there are many people who might be skeptical of it, yet it has been a part of ancient Chinese medicine (used by Taoists) for thousands of years.

In recent years, it has been shown that no number of crunches will magically melt those few extra pounds that you carry around your midsection. Mostly because stomach or belly fat is always the last place for the weight to go from, because its where the cortisol factor lies (discussed earlier). So, this simple massage exercise provides a method that will help to clean and detoxify (as well as also helping to melt away fat).

A more recent study published inside the Journal of the European Academy of Dermatology and Venereology (2010) concluded that lymphatic drainage massage, connective tissue manipulation, and the use of mechanical massage helped to decrease fat; the thickness of the fat underneath the skin. The average was 2 millimeters. In addition, having a stomach massage can help speed the passage of foods consumed through your digestive tract. Also aiding constipation, according to a publication in the Journal of Bodywork and Movement Therapies (2011).

How Does It Work?

This Chinese medicine in the form of massage uses exercise to improve the internal digestive system while increasing the body's capability of detoxifying itself and eliminating waste as a necessity. On top of the immediate effects, the following benefits are gained:

- Aid in detoxifying the intestines
- Relieves the effects of constipation
- Helps stimulate internal organs in your abdominal region
- Help melt adipose tissues
- Helps improve the body's circulation in the abdominal area
- Aids in eliminating conditions such as indigestion, vomiting, and nausea

How to Do the Exercise

1. Lie on your back. Make sure the surface is firm, and your back is flat.
2. Warm your hands by rubbing them together briskly.
3. Place one hand flat on your belly button (navel).
4. Apply firm (not hard) pressure with your hand.
5. Start rubbing in small, clockwise circles around your belly button.
6. Slowly expand the size of the circles you complete as your hand moves outward on your stomach.
7. Once your hand has reached the extreme part of your stomach, you can reverse the direction and decrease the size of the circles as you gently rub until your hand is back on your belly button. Now, you'll go anti-clockwise.
8. This only takes a few minutes to complete, and until your hand reaches the extreme of your stomach. It easily returns

back to your belly button. This can be done twice per day or as often as required.

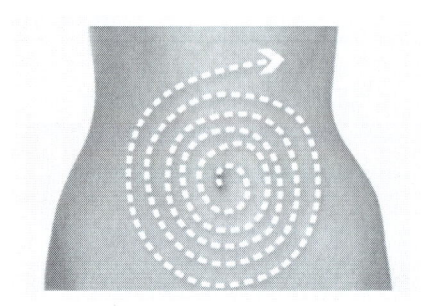

Does It Work?

Many people disregard this massage technique as a gimmick. Here are two individuals who it helped. These are valid case studies from people who had become disillusioned with most other means of weight loss.

A fifty-five-year-old bank president who was overweight. This man always felt sluggish and was heavily constipated. It was his secretary who advised he should try the exercise because he had nothing else to lose.

Once he had performed the massage exercise, he finally resolved his constipation issue and regulated his bowels. Not only did he lose forty pounds from doing the exercise on a "religious" basis, he also became full of newfound energy that he hadn't experienced before.

The second case was a twenty-nine-year-old woman who approached after a lecture. At the time, she was size eighteen and was worried she would never lose her excess inches. After having the exercise explained to her, she was unsure that she would be able to stick to doing it. However, once she had been shown how simple and fun it was, she gave it a go.

After a two-week period of performing the massage, her size eighteen dress that used to be tight, now started to become loose! With maintaining the massage exercise, she eventually reached a size eleven.

These examples show how this rubbing exercise can give results when it comes to breaking up fatty build up in the abdominal region. These can then be expelled from the body by natural means. The ancient practice is well-worth exploring. And it worked for me! I lost over a hundred pounds!

It is not magic, and it is based on a thousand-year-old practice. It does appear that fat is magically rubbed away from the stomach!! If it works, then "Voila!"

Chapter Nine
BOOST THE LOSS WITH BIKE RIDING

When it comes to losing a few extra pounds around the waist, there is quite a lot to consider to truly get rid of the stubborn ones. Especially those that seem to linger, no matter what you do to get rid of them.

The consensus has always been more exercise and specific exercises that are geared to removing belly fat. If things were that simple, maybe that small podge would have disappeared already, **but the body doesn't quite work in that way.**

More Exercise

We know to lose a pound in weight equates to 3500 calories, which need to be burned. Doing this through exercise alone, means you need excessive workouts for around four hours per day. This would, over time, do more harm than good. You would be working out so much that all your lean muscle mass would be consumed by energy, and well before those pounds were shifted from your stomach.

Actually, the harder you train, the harder the body will try and keep those pounds wrapped around your waist. The body can do this by moving fat from other areas, and as was mentioned earlier, this is why they are the last few pounds that are usually removed.

Less Exercise

When it comes to fat and the burning of it, the process can quickly become complicated, and the way that many people are informed of the best way to do it is, unfortunately, a little misleading.

Rather than working out excessively, **it is more beneficial when you combine your calorie deficit with exercise that uses more muscles, and thus enables you to burn more calories.**

Earlier, we saw that your calorie deficit per day would equate to a loss of between one to two pounds in weight that you can utilize naturally. When you introduce exercise into your program, you can burn many more calories.

The problem with too much exercise is, your body becomes accustomed to this rigorous regime and suffers from workout stress, as well building muscle. A couple of things that are never mentioned with muscle building are, it is heavier than fat, so if you increase muscle mass, you will get heavier, and secondly, you will not see the definition with any muscle you have gained until the fat has gone. The simple reason being, you cannot turn fat into muscle, it is two, entirely, different things.

Bike Riding to Lose Real Belly Fat

When you take up bike riding as your primary form of exercise, you can lose these stubborn waist inches much more comfortably and much quicker, too. This is down to the fact that you are not focusing on one muscle group.

In truth, you use many more muscles in the body when riding a bike for around 30 minutes per day than you would in a gym, and **this means all of your body starts working to burn these excess calories,** and that includes your stomach.

How Many Calories Can You Burn?

Without taking into account a person's exact body weight, and the pace that they peddle. Let's see. Over a period of thirty minutes on a stationary bike, the following can be achieved:

Moderate intensity for a 185-lb. person can burn **300** calories.

High intensity for a 185-lb. person can burn **466** calories.

If you take your bike riding outdoors the following calories burned can be:

Cycling at **15 mph for 30 minutes,** a 185-lb. person can burn **444** calories.

Raise the speed up to **19 mph for 30 minutes,** and a 185-lb person can burn **533** calories.

Once you get over **20mph for 30 minutes,** you can burn over **700** calories for a 185-lb. person.

If anyone tells you that you can lose fat from one part of the body (and this is what you target), they are definitely wrong. You will gain muscle in that area, and, it is only when you have lost overall bodyweight that you will see the muscles underneath. Good to know!

Chapter Ten

EIGHT GREAT GREEN SMOOTHIE RECIPES FOR YOU TO ENJOY!

Juicing makes me feel amazing. I noticed an immediate increase in my energy levels, and I had more regular bowel movements too. I don't know that I could live without juicing now. The tastes are unbelievable, the energy boost is second-to-none, and the fun of juicing is definitely worth it! And… it's so easy!

The benefits of juicing include: being able to measure your drink consumption in cups, detoxification, a source of nutrients from multiple fruits and vegetables, energy boosting capability, the ease of getting all your needs in one drink, and the capability of adaptation to mealtimes, or as a meal replacement.

In addition, juicing is fantastic because the foods are broken down allowing for easier digestion by the stomach, which doesn't need to use the energy it usually would to break it down. I absolutely love juicing!

RECIPE #1: COCONUT SPINACH: INGREDIENT LIST:

- 1 1/2 oz. of baby spinach
- 1 banana - peeled
- 1 squash - chopped
- 1 teaspoon of cinnamon
- 4 tablespoons of walnuts
- 1 cup of coconut water
- 1 cup of ice

Directions:

When ready, simply process all the ingredients together in your favorite blender. You can shake it up or stir it up, then serve and enjoy. Cube or chop vegetables to make them blitz easier before blending. I like to add any leafy vegetables in last, and then add a touch more water if I want the consistency smoother or silkier. Great garnishes include: lemon, celery, chia seeds, or a slice of tomato. Add ice on a hot day to make the drink cooler.

RECIPE #2: BUTTERNUT-SPINACH SQUASH: INGREDIENT LIST:

- 1 1/2 oz. of baby spinach
- 1 banana - peeled
- 4 oz. butternut squash
- 1 teaspoon of matcha powder
- 1 tablespoon of hemp seeds
- 1 cup of water
- 1 cup ice

Directions:

When ready, simply process all the ingredients together in your favorite blender. You can shake it up or stir it up, then serve and enjoy. Cube or chop vegetables to make them blitz easier before blending. I like to add any leafy vegetables in last, and then add a touch more water if I want the consistency smoother or silkier. Great garnishes include: lemon, celery, chia seeds, or a slice of tomato. Add ice on a hot day to make the drink cooler.

RECIPE #3: LUXURY LUCUMA: INGREDIENT LIST:

- 1 1/2 oz. of baby spinach
- 1 orange - peeled
- 1 pear - chopped
- 1 teaspoon of lucuma
- 1 tablespoon of chia seeds
- 1 cup of water
- 1 cup of ice

Directions:

When ready, simply process all the ingredients together in your favorite blender. You can shake it up or stir it up, then serve and enjoy. Cube or chop vegetables to make them blitz easier before blending. I like to add any leafy vegetables in last, and then add a touch more water if I want the consistency smoother or silkier. Great garnishes include: lemon, celery, chia seeds, or a slice of tomato. Add ice on a hot day to make the drink cooler.

RECIPE #4: APPLE PECAN PARADISE: INGREDIENT LIST:

- 1 1/2 oz. of baby spinach
- 1 banana - peeled
- 1 container of cinnamon applesauce - (1/2 cup)
- 1 tablespoon of oats
- 3 tablespoons of pecans
- 1 cup of water
- 1 cup of ice

Directions:

When ready, simply process all the ingredients together in your favorite blender. You can shake it up or stir it up, then serve and enjoy. Cube or chop vegetables to make them blitz easier before blending. I like to add any leafy vegetables in last, and then add a touch more water if I want the consistency smoother or silkier. Great garnishes include: lemon, celery, chia seeds, or a slice of tomato. Add ice on a hot day to make the drink cooler.

RECIPE #5: GOJI GO-GO: INGREDIENT LIST:

- 1 1/2 oz. of baby spinach
- 1 apple - chopped
- 1 banana - peeled
- 1 tablespoon of goji berries
- 1 tablespoon of flaxseeds
- 1 cup of water
- 1 cup of ice

Directions:

When ready, simply process all the ingredients together in your favorite blender. You can shake it up or stir it up, then serve and enjoy. Cube or chop vegetables to make them blitz easier before blending. I like to add any leafy vegetables in last, and then add a touch more water if I want the consistency smoother or silkier. Great garnishes include: lemon, celery, chia seeds, or a slice of tomato. Add ice on a hot day to make the drink cooler.

RECIPE #6: PERSIMMON-MINT MAGIC: INGREDIENT LIST:

- 1 1/2 oz. of collard greens
- 1 apple - chopped
- 1 persimmon - topped

- 3 sprigs of mint
- 1 teaspoon of matcha tea
- 1 cup of water
- 1 cup of ice

Directions:

When ready, simply process all the ingredients together in your favorite blender. You can shake it up or stir it up, then serve and enjoy. Cube or chop vegetables to make them blitz easier before blending. I like to add any leafy vegetables in last, and then add a touch more water if I want the consistency smoother or silkier. Great garnishes include: lemon, celery, chia seeds, or a slice of tomato. Add ice on a hot day to make the drink cooler.

RECIPE #7: PEARS N' SPINACH: INGREDIENT LIST:

- 1 1/2 oz. of baby spinach
- 1 apple - chopped
- 1 pear - chopped
- 1 teaspoon of cinnamon
- 1 tablespoon of flaxseeds
- 1 cup of water
- 1 cup of ice

Directions:

When ready, simply process all the ingredients together in your favorite blender. You can shake it up or stir it up, then serve and enjoy. Cube or chop vegetables to make them blitz easier before blending. I like to add any leafy vegetables in last, and then add a touch more water if I want the consistency smoother or silkier. Great garnishes include: lemon, celery, chia seeds, or a slice of tomato. Add ice on a hot day to make the drink cooler.

RECIPE #8: THE LIMEY GRAPE: INGREDIENT LIST:

- 1 1/2 oz. of collard greens
- 4 oz. of grapes
- 2 mini cucumbers - chopped
- 1 lime - juiced
- 1 tablespoon of chia seeds
- 1 cup of ice
- 1 cup of water

Directions:

When ready, simply process all the ingredients together in your favorite blender. You can shake it up or stir it up, then serve and enjoy. Cube or chop vegetables to make them blitz easier before blending. I like to add any leafy vegetables in last, and then add a touch more water if I want the consistency smoother or silkier. Great garnishes include: lemon, celery, chia seeds, or a slice of tomato. Add ice on a hot day to make the drink cooler.

IN CONCLUSION

Thanks so much for joining me here. **Remember to stay positive** and keep your eye on the prize as you take the steps toward success. I absolutely love that you're taking your health into your own hands. Your health always needs to be the priority. **Always act safely and responsibly,** and make sure that you get **plenty of sleep** each night. Anything that helps with stress relief is great, too. I highly recommend meditation and yoga, if you enjoy these modalities. Even a "nana nap" for 20 minutes can do the world of good!

If you can plan ahead in terms of meal preparation, meal times, and exercise times, then you can get to your end goal faster, and because you are organized and willing to make the change, it WILL happen for you.

Remember, **I am here cheering you on**, and my thoughts and my heart are with you all the way. I know you've totally got this!

I am sending you so much love and luck on your amazing journey. Keep going, because I am here with you - all the way! Well done! And I'm sending loads of love to you.

Stay positive; always, lots of love from Emma xx

Remember, if you haven't already read my title, "How I Lost 100 Pounds! My Personal Weight Loss Strategies for Optimum Happiness," make sure you get your FREE copy today. Inside you'll learn exactly how I lost my weight, and the benefits of knowing the must-do nutrition, and other amazing secrets including myths, water weight, the only exercise you really need, the ancient and easy technique to help slim you quickly, how to balance meals, and much, much more! I hope you love it. It's my very special gift to you!

Made in United States
North Haven, CT
25 November 2021